21-day Challenge

21-day Challenge

Low-impact Exercise

Reneé A. George

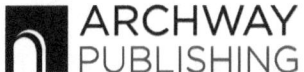

Exercise 4 Life LLC

◤ ARCHWAY
PUBLISHING

Archway Publishing books may be ordered through booksellers or by contacting:

Archway Publishing
1663 Liberty Drive
Bloomington, IN 47403
www.archwaypublishing.com
1 (888) 242-5904

Edited by Mrs. Lorena Finger and Ms. Janelle Finger.

Scripture taken from the New King James Version®. Copyright © 1982 by Thomas Nelson. Used by permission. All rights reserved.

ISBN: 978-1-4808-7935-5 (sc)
ISBN: 978-1-4808-7937-9 (hc)
ISBN: 978-1-4808-7936-2 (e)

Library of Congress Control Number: 2019911460

Print information available on the last page.

Archway Publishing rev. date: 9/4/2019

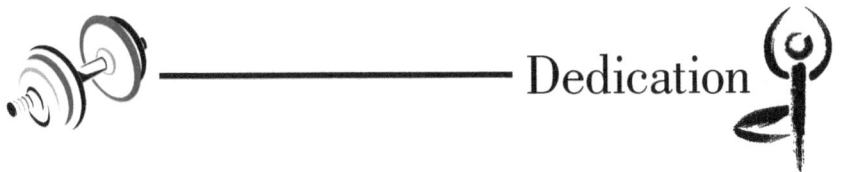

Dedication

I would like to give thanks to my Lord Jesus Christ who has giving me the ability to finish this book. A Big thank you to <u>All</u> who help me in anyway, A special Thank you to Antoinette Benitez, Shyann Morton, Lorena Fingers, Janelle Fingers, Justin George, Shan and my Uncle Sterling

Thank you all for your time help and Patience, I wouldn't have made it without all of you.

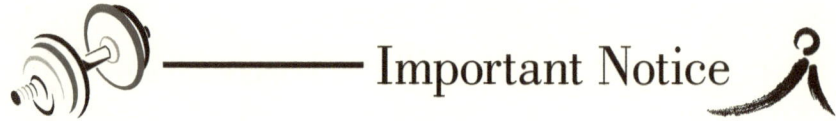# Important Notice

This program guide is a product of Exercise 4 Life and is not for reproduction of any kind. This book may be purchased online or at exercise4lifellc.777@gmail.com.

Seven Tips for Your Healthy Lifestyle

1. Consult your doctor before doing any exercise program, get regular checkups.
2. Eat balanced meals and in moderation; increase your intake of vegetables and fruits.
3. Drink plenty of water, stay properly hydrated.
4. Get plenty of rest.
5. Be consistent.
6. Have lots of fun.
7. Track your progress.

— Something from Nay

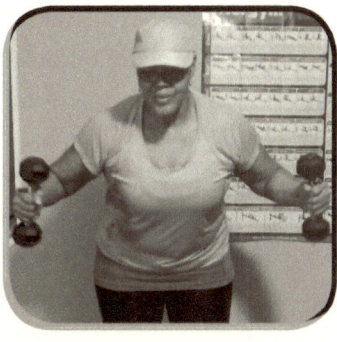

Hello! Congratulations on reading this book. I have a very big smile on my face and so much joy inside because of the journey you are about to go on. At times, it will be hard for some and easy for others. You might not feel up to it on some days, or you might say, "I just don't have time for this." If you don't like exercise, think, *I can do this.* Just take baby steps. Work your way up to the next level. Have fun with it! All you will need is your body, a chair, and some music. Put your music on, and let's do this! I say this because I know you can do it. I'm physically challenged due to a car accident. I love music, dancing, and exercise. Remember this: Never ever give up on you and your dreams!

These twenty-one-day low-impact exercise challenges are dedicated to myself especially because I have some physically challenges. But all are welcome. Beginners and adults, let's do this!

Know who you are,
Where you came from,
Where you are going.
Never ever give up on you and your dreams!

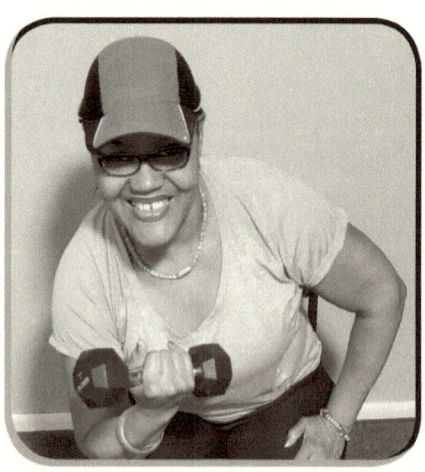

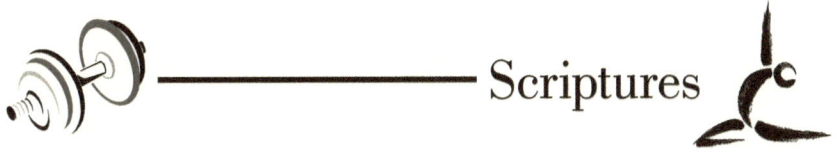# Scriptures

2 Timothy 1:7

> *For God has not given us a spirit of fear, but of power and of love and a sound mind*

Ephesians 6:11

> *Put on the whole armor of God, that you may be able to stand against the wiles of the devil*

Romans 8:28

> *And we know that all things work together for good to those who love God, to those who are the called according to His purpose*

Jeremiah 29 11:14

> *11 For I know the thoughts that I think toward you, says the Lord, thoughts of peace and not of evil, to give you a future and a hope*

> *12 Then you will call upon Me and go and Pray to me, and I will listen to you.*

> *13 And you will seek Me and find me, when you search for Me with all your heart*

14 I will be found by you, says the LORD, and I will bring you back from your captivity: I will gather you from all the nations and from all the places where I have driven you, Says the LORD, and I will bring you to the place from which I cause you to be carried away captive.

The reason I picked these scriptures was because the pain I endured was so indescribable. The challenges that I went through during my healing period were very hard for me to overcome. I felt like giving up, but I didn't. I cried so much. I cried out to the Lord Jesus Christ to please help. I still need and have much more work to do, but Jesus has me—and all of us—here for a reason. We must do our best to never ever give up because He has our back. His hands are bigger than our hands. He will never leave you nor forsake you.

Before you do these low-impact exercises, remember to consult your doctor. Drink plenty of water. Always go at your own pace. All exercises can be modified. If you need to slow down or take a break, do so. It is also very important to listen to your body. Your eating habits and nutrition are also very important. It is 80 percent diet and 20 percent exercise.

Below, you will see a calorie guide that I used. You may use it as well or not, but remember to consult your doctor first, especially if you have health problems or are on medication. And have fun!

Breakfast, Lunch, Dinner, and Snack: Pick Your Number of Calories per Meal★★★

1,300 Calories		*1,600 Calories*		*1,800 Calories*	
Breakfast	300	Breakfast	385	Breakfast	475
Lunch	400	Lunch	580	Lunch	625
Dinner	450	Lunch	485	Dinner	550
Snack	150	Snack	150	Snack	150

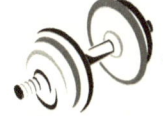 ———————— Fitness Test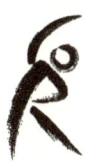

Name: _____

Date Started: _____

Age: _____

	Begin	Halfway	Finished
Balance:	_____	_____	_____
Flexibility:	_____	_____	_____

You can sit in a chair or on the floor for the toe touch **********

Each exercise below will be done for thirty to forty-five seconds.

1. Sit to Stand   _____ _____ _____
2. Seated Squats   _____ _____ _____
3. Roll Shoulder Backward   _____ _____ _____
4. Pull Down   _____ _____ _____
5. Arm Side Stretch   _____ _____ _____

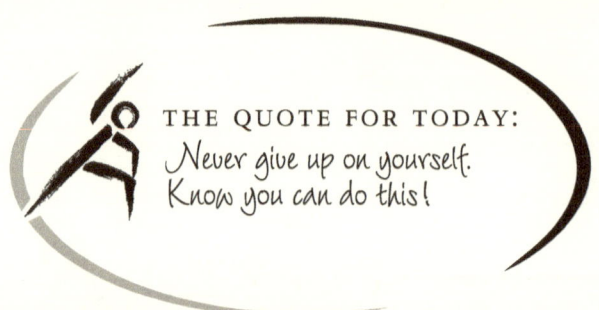

THE QUOTE FOR TODAY:
Never give up on yourself.
Know you can do this!

Day 1

Each morning, midday, and evening exercise will be forty-five seconds and then rest for fifteen seconds. Always warm up before exercise and cool down after exercise.

☀ Morning: Stretching Upper Body

1. Upper-body shoulder rotation
2. Pull down
3. Biceps: Target the upper body, underarm, shoulder.
4. Squats: Do twenty-five. If this is too much for you to start off with, do what you can. It's okay.

🌤 Midday: Chair and Stretching Exercises

1. Leg raises
2. Toe raises
3. Knee raises
4. Squats—twenty-five

🌙 Evening: Stretching and Lower-Body, Toning Front and Back of the Thighs Exercises

1. Hip bridge
2. Single-leg circle
3. Standing crossover toe touches
4. Squats—twenty-five.

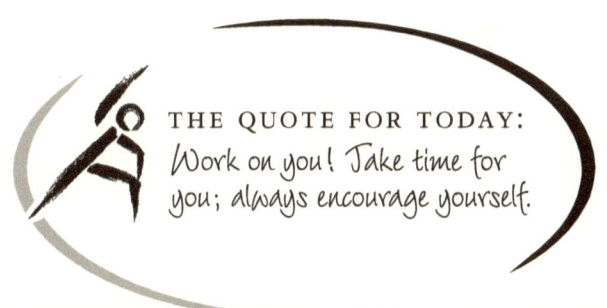

Day 2

☀ Morning: Stretching and Upper-Body Exercises

1. Sideways hands bound
2. Seated forward bend
3. Beginning back bend
4. Squats—twenty-five

☀ Midday: Stretching and Chair Exercises

1. Sit to stand
2. Seated sit-ups for the abs and core
3. Seated squat lunges for the thighs and butt
4. Squats—twenty-five

☾ Evening: Stretching and Lower-Body Exercises

1. Lying side jacks
2. Cobra to child pose
3. Sideways easy pose
4. Squats—Twenty-five

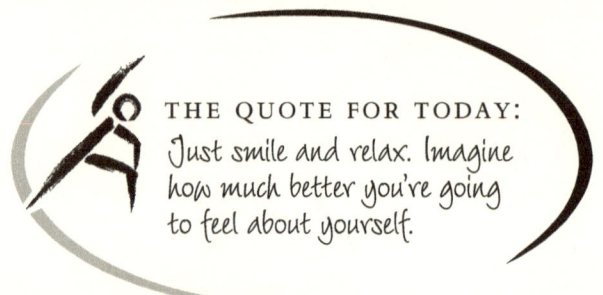

Day 3

☀ Morning: Stretching for Upper Body

1. Plank pose
2. Half shoulder stand
3. Hips raised, extended
4. Squats

🌤 Midday: Stretching and Chair Exercises

1. Knee to elbow lifts
2. Bending
3. Single knee lifts
4. Squats

🌙 Evening: Stretching and Exercises

1. Knee to chest lifts
2. Body bent to right side and left side with hands behind your head
3. Hips raised, extended
4. Squats

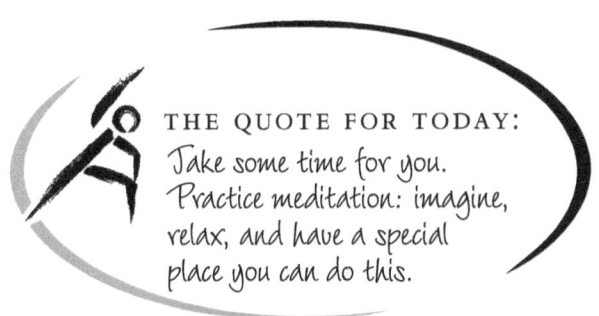

Day 4

☀ Morning: Stretching and Upper-Body Exercises

1. Sideways pose
2. Half-upward stretch
3. Big toe touch
4. Squats

🌄 Midday: Stretching and Chair Exercises

1. Knee to elbow lifts
2. Seated sit-ups for the abs, core
3. Sit to stand
4. Squats

🌙 Evening: Stretching and Lower-Body Exercises

1. Lying side jacks
2. Child pose
3. Blend stretch
4. Squats

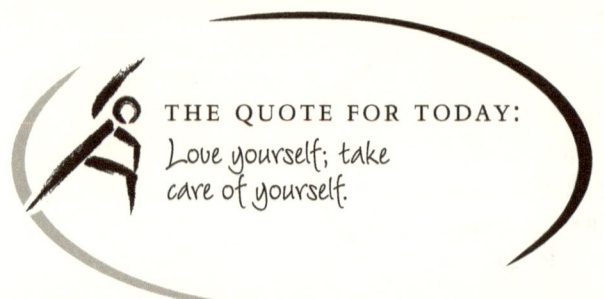

Day 5

☀ **Morning: Upper-Body Stretching, Shoulder Rotation Targeting the Upper Under Arm, Shoulder, Biceps**

1. Arm side stretch
2. Pull down
3. Arm circles
4. Squats

🌄 **Midday: Stretching and Chair Exercises**

1. Side body stretch
2. Roll shoulder backward
3. Sit to stand
4. Squats

🌙 **Evening: Stretching and Exercises**

1. Child pose
2. Back stretch
3. Lying side jacks
4. Squats

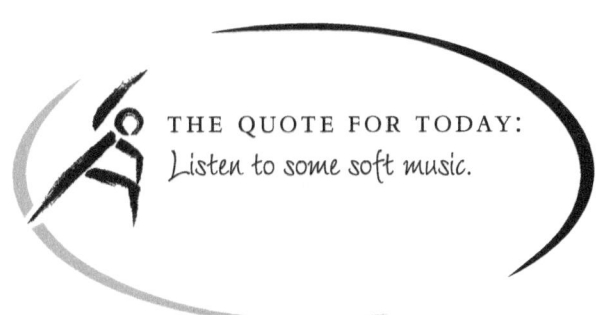

Day 6

☀ Morning: Stretching for Upper Body

1. Arm side stretch
2. Pull down
3. Arm circles
4. Squats

🌅 Midday: Stretching and Chair Exercises

1. Shoulder squeeze
2. Wall push-ups, both arms and hands
3. Hip flexion, left leg/right leg
4. Seated chair squats

🌙 Evening: Stretching and Exercises

1. Superman: Hold position for forty-five seconds. If that's too much, it's okay. Do your best.
2. Hip bridge
3. Knee raises, left knee/right knee
4. Squats

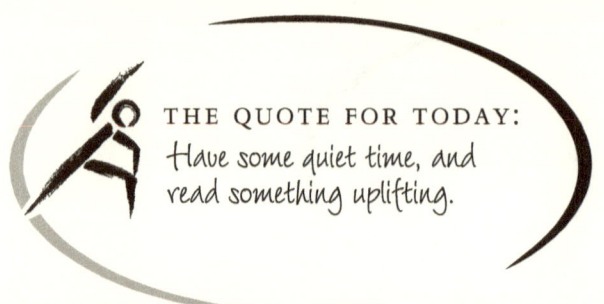

Day 7

☀ Morning: Upper-Body Stretching

1. Arm side stretching
2. Pull down
3. Arm circles
4. Squats

🌄 Midday: Stretching and Chair Exercises

1. Shoulder squeeze
2. Wall push-ups, both arms and hands
3. Hip flexion, left leg/right leg
4. Seated chair squats

🌙 Evening: Stretching and Exercises

1. Superman: Hold position for forty-five seconds. If that's too much, it's okay. Do your best.
2. Hip bridge
3. Knee raises, left knee/right knee
4. Squats

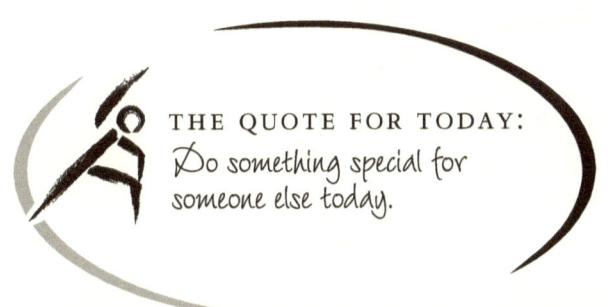

Day 8

☀ Morning: Stretching and Exercises

1. Arm side stretch
2. Pull down
3. Arm circles
4. Squats

⛅ Midday: Stretching and Chair Exercises

1. Shoulder squeeze
2. Wall push-ups, both arms and hands
3. Hip flexion, left leg/right leg
4. Seated chair squats

☾ Evening: Stretching and Exercises

1. Superman: Hold position for forty-five seconds. If that's too much, it's okay. Do your best.
2. Hip bridge
3. Knee raises, left knee/right knee
4. Squats

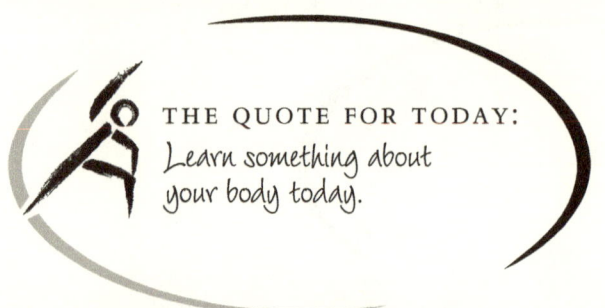

THE QUOTE FOR TODAY:
*Learn something about
your body today.*

Day 9

☀ Morning: Upper-Body Stretch

1. Arm side stretch
2. Pull down
3. Arm circles
4. Squats

⛅ Midday: Chair Stretching and Exercises

1. Shoulder squeeze
2. Wall push-ups, both arms and hands
3. Hip flexion, left leg/right leg
4. Seated chair squats

☾ Evening: Stretching and Exercises

1. Superman: Hold position for forty-five seconds. If that's too much, it's okay. Do your best.
2. Hip bridge
3. Knee raises, left knee/right knee
4. Squats

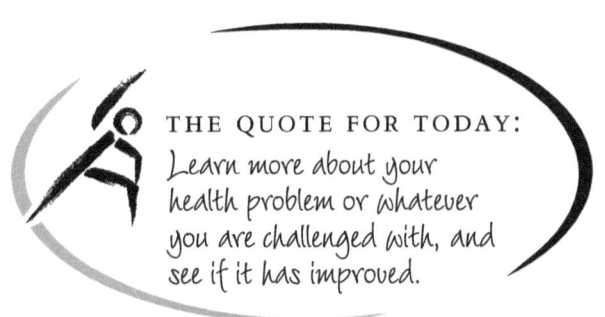

Day 10

☀ Morning: Upper-Body Stretching

1. Arm side stretch
2. Pull down
3. Arm circles
4. Squats

🌄 Midday: Stretching and Chair Exercises

1. Shoulder squeeze
2. Wall push-ups, both arms and hands
3. Hip flexion, left leg/right leg
4. Seated chair squats

🌙 Evening: Stretching and Exercises

1. Superman: Hold position for forty-five seconds. If that's too much, it's okay. Do your best.
2. Hip bridge
3. Knee raises, left knee/right knee
4. Squats

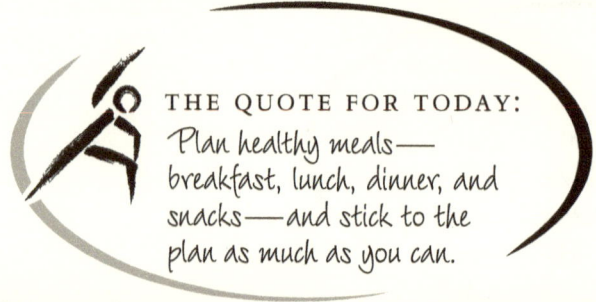

Day 11

☀ Morning: Upper-Body Stretching

1. Sideways hands bound (shoulder) standing poses (yoga)
2. Forward bend (yoga)
3. Seated forward bend
4. Squats

⛅ Midday: Stretching and Chair Exercises

1. Side twist
2. Jumping jacks
3. Heel lifts
4. Squats

☾ Evening: Stretching and Exercises

1. Plank (core)
2. Hip crossover (core)
3. Cycling Russian twist (core)
4. Squats

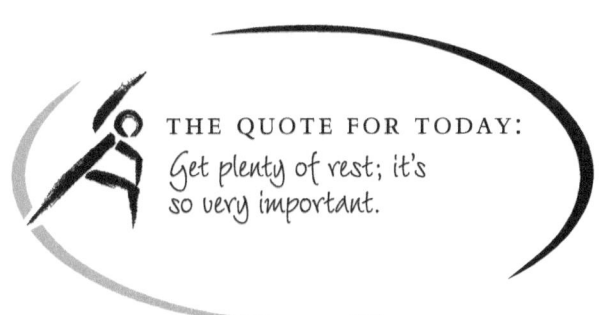

Day 12

☀ Morning: Stretching

1. Sideway hands bound (shoulders) standing pose (yoga)
2. Forward bend (yoga)
3. Seated forward bend
4. Squats

🌄 Midday: Stretching and Chair Exercises

1. Side twist
2. Jumping jacks
3. Heel lifts
4. Overhead triceps extension
5. Squats

🌙 Evening: Stretching and Exercises

1. Sit-ups (core)
2. Side crunch (core)
3. Side bend (core)
4. Push-ups (chest)
5. Squats

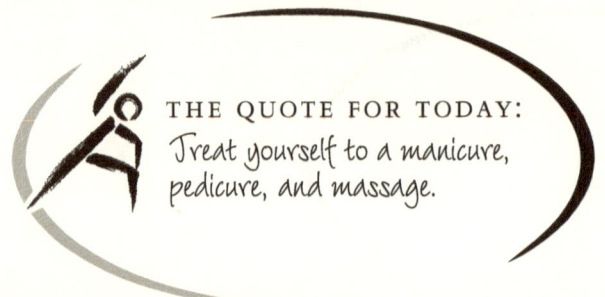

Treat yourself to a manicure, pedicure, and massage.

Day 13

☀ Morning: Stretching

1. Sideways hands bound (shoulders) (yoga)
2. Forward blend (yoga)
3. Seated forward bend
4. Squats

☀ Midday: Stretching and Chair Exercises

1. Side twist
2. Jumping jacks
3. Heel lifts
4. Overhead triceps extension
5. Squats

☾ Evening: Stretching and Exercises

1. Plank (core)
2. Hip crossover (core)
3. Cycling Russian twist (core)
4. Alternating shoulder press and twist
5. Squats

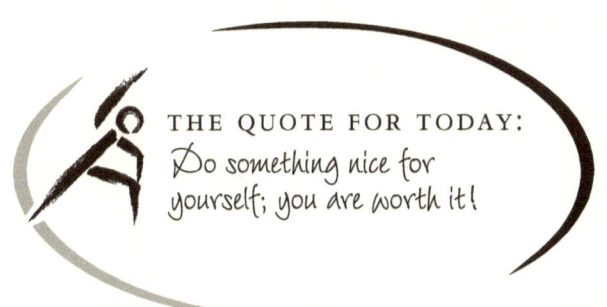

Day 14

☀ Morning: Stretching

1. Sideways hands bound (standing pose) (yoga)
2. Forward bend (yoga)
3. Seated forward bend
4. Squats

🌄 Midday: Stretching and Chair Exercises

1. Side twist
2. Jumping jacks
3. Squats
4. Overhead triceps extension

🌙 Evening: Stretching and Exercises

1. Plank (core)
2. Hip crossover (core)
3. Cycling Russian twist (core)
4. Squats
5. Alternating shoulder press and twist

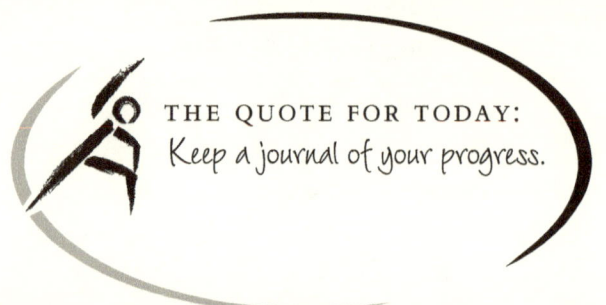

Day 15

☀ Morning: Stretching

1. Sideways hands bound (shoulders) standing pose (yoga)
2. Forward bend (yoga)
3. Seated forward bend
4. Squats

🌄 Midday: Stretching and Chair Exercises

1. Side twist
2. Jumping jacks
3. Heel lifts
4. Squats
5. Overhead triceps extension

🌙 Evening: Stretching and Exercises

1. Plank (core)
2. Hip crossover (core)
3. Cycling Russian twist (core)
4. Squats
5. Overhead triceps extension

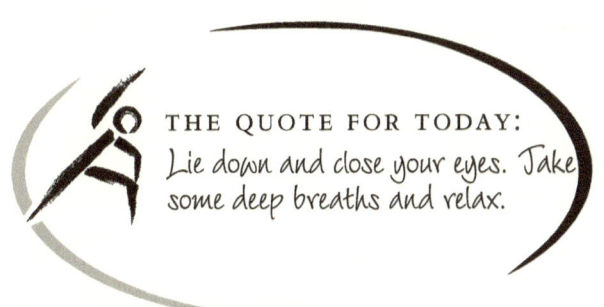

Day 16

☀ Morning: Stretching

1. Arm side stretch
2. Pull down
3. Arm circles
4. Squats

🌅 Midday: Stretching and Chair Exercises

1. Toe lifts
2. Seated squat lunges
3. Seated sit-ups
4. Chair squats
5. Overhead triceps extension

🌙 Evening: Stretching and Exercises

1. Sit-ups (core)
2. Side crunch (core)
3. Side bends (core)
4. Squats
5. Push-ups (chest)

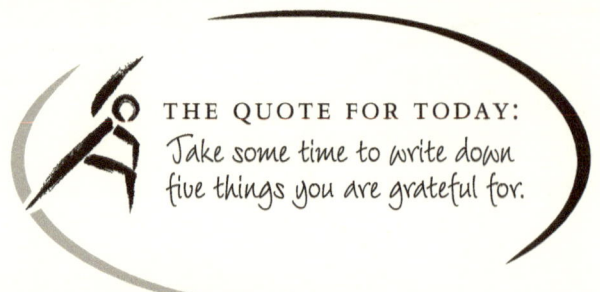

Day 17

☀ Morning: Stretching

1. Arm side stretch
2. Pull down
3. Arm circles
4. Squats

⛅ Midday: Stretching and Chair Exercises

1. Toe lifts
2. Seated sit-ups
3. Chair squats
4. Seated squat lunges
5. Overhead triceps extension

☾ Evening: Stretching and Exercises

1. Sit-ups (core)
2. Side crunch (core)
3. Side bend (core)
4. Squats
5. Push-ups (Chest)

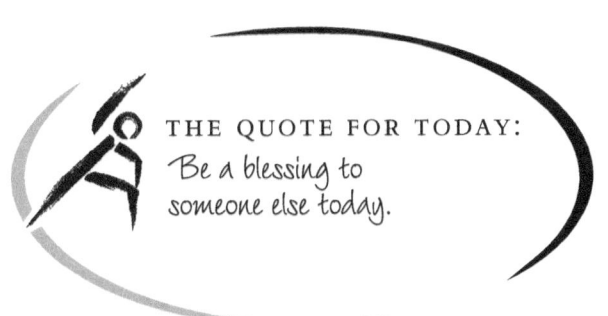

THE QUOTE FOR TODAY:
*Be a blessing to
someone else today.*

Day 18

☀ Morning: Stretching

1. Arm side stretch
2. Pull down
3. Arm circles
4. Squats

⛅ Midday: Stretching and Chair Exercises

1. Toe lifts
2. Seated squat lunges
3. Chair squats
4. Overhead triceps extension

☾ Evening: Stretching and Exercises

1. Sit-ups (core)
2. Side crunch (core)
3. Side bend (core)
4. Squats
5. Push-ups (chest)

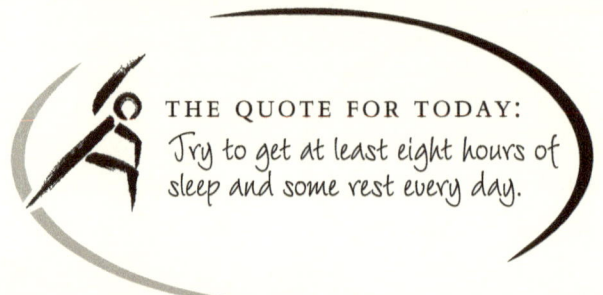

Day 19

☀ Morning: Stretching

1. Arm side stretch
2. Pull down
3. Arm circles
4. Squats

⛅ Midday: Stretching and Chair Exercises

1. Toe lifts
2. Seated squat lunges
3. Seated sit-ups
4. Chair squats
5. Overhead triceps extension

🌙 Evening: Stretching and Exercises

1. Sit ups (core)
2. Side crunch (core)
3. Side bend (core)
4. Squats
5. Push-ups (chest)

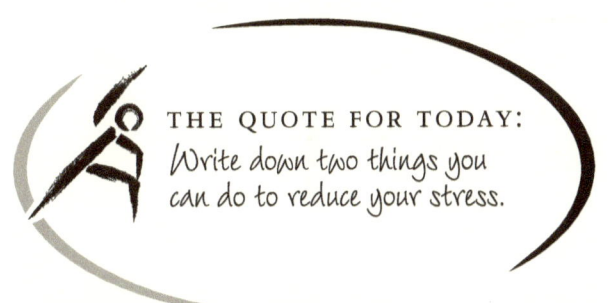

THE QUOTE FOR TODAY:
*Write down two things you
can do to reduce your stress.*

Day 20

☀ Morning: Stretching

1. Arm side stretching
2. Pull down
3. Arm circles
4. Squats

☀ Midday: Stretching and Chair Exercises

1. Toe lifts
2. Seated squat lunges
3. Seated sit-ups
4. Chair squats
5. Overhead triceps extension

☽ Evenings: Stretching and Exercises

1. Sit-ups (core)
2. Side crunch (core)
3. Side bend (core)
4. Squats
5. Overhead triceps extension

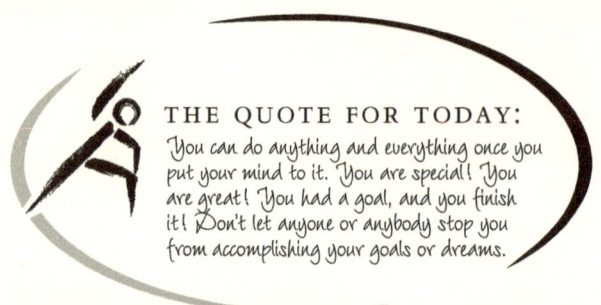

Day 21

☀ Morning: Stretching, and Let's Thank the Lord Jesus Christ that You Made It

Today is your last day! Let's have some fun. Just put some music on and dance.

⛅ Midday:

Let's put on some soft or quiet music, so you can meditate on how you are going to the next level and how you love your body. From this day forward, you are going to take time out to take care of this temple that God has giving you.

☾ Evening: Stretching and Yoga

Excellent!

Give yourself a big hug and a smile. You did it! Now do something really nice and special for yourself. It doesn't matter how small or big it is. Just do it.

Congratulations!

You have finished the twenty-one-day challenge. How do you feel? Excellent, great, wonderful, all right? Just know exercise is for everyone. It keeps you healthy inside and out. So keep up the good work, have fun with it, and enjoy taking care of yourself and your body. You only have one! When you look at yourself and see what you have accomplished, just smile and say, "I am special! Thank you, Jesus!"

Remember, never give up on yourself!

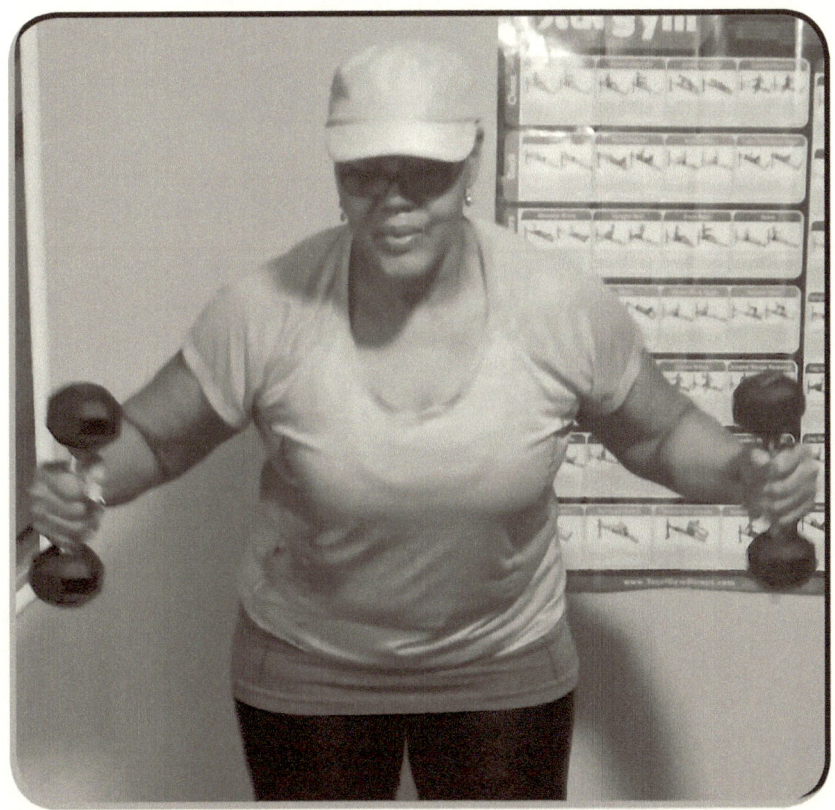

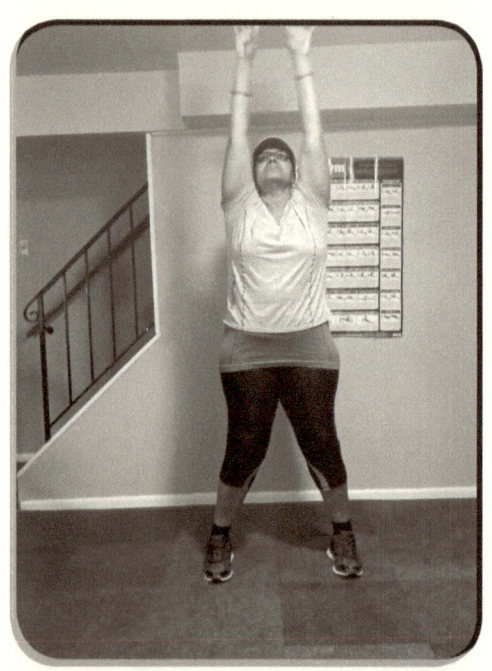

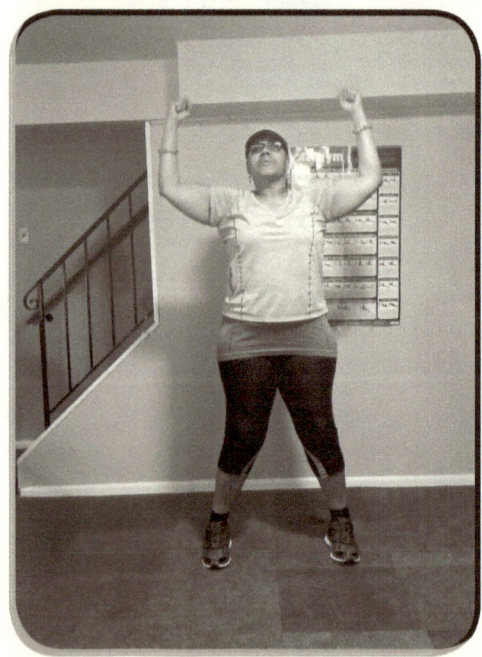

Pull down

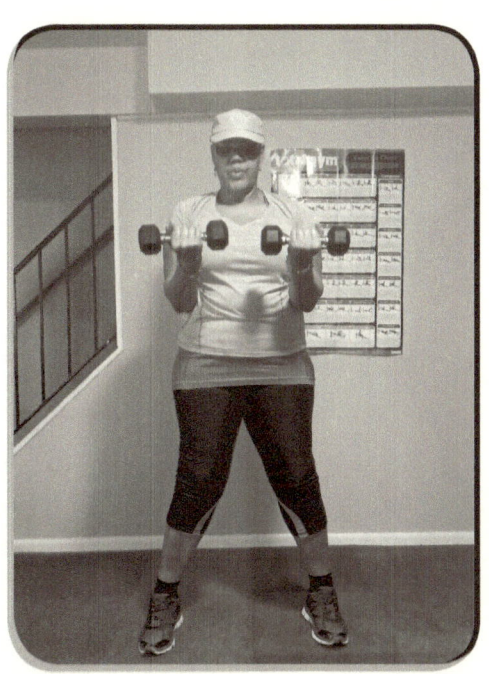

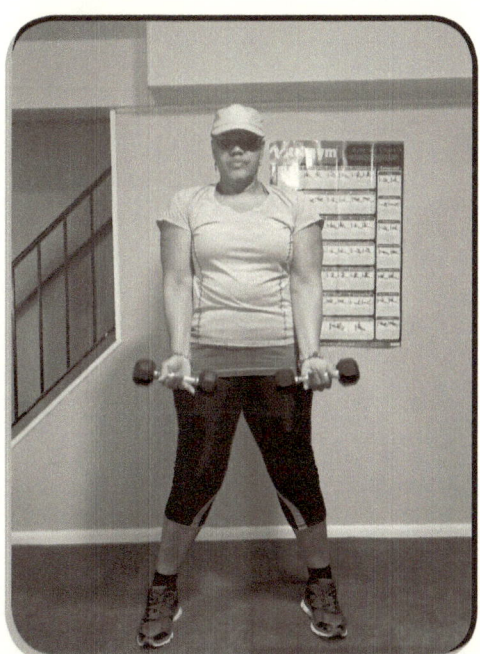

Biceps: Target the upper body

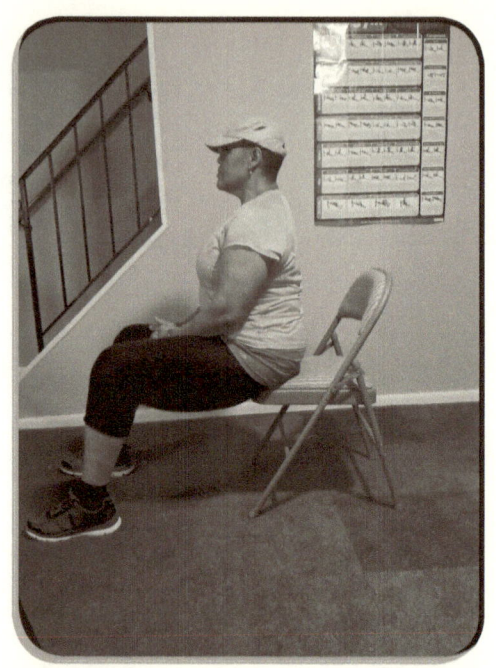

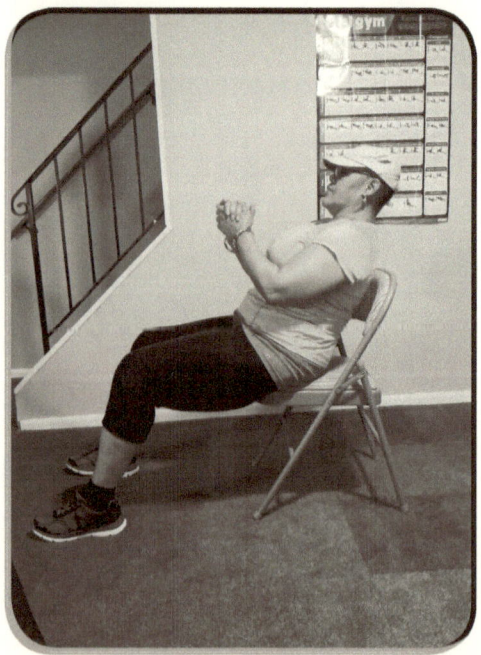

Seated sit-ups

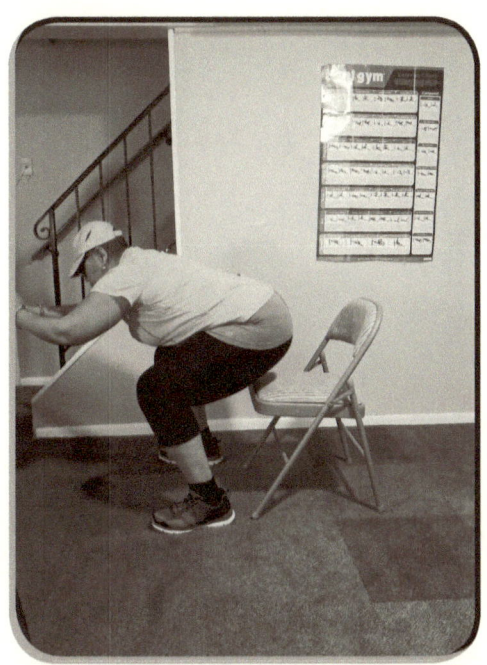

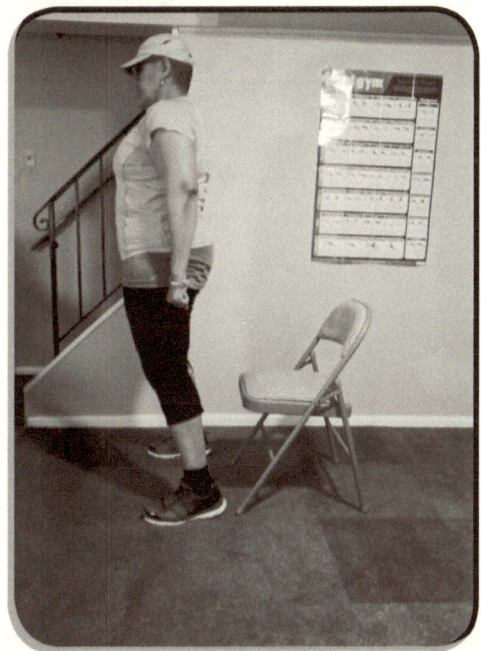

Sit -to- Stand

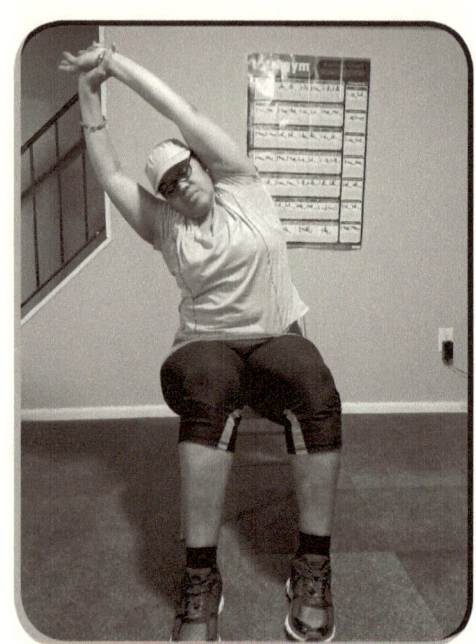

Sideways hand bound

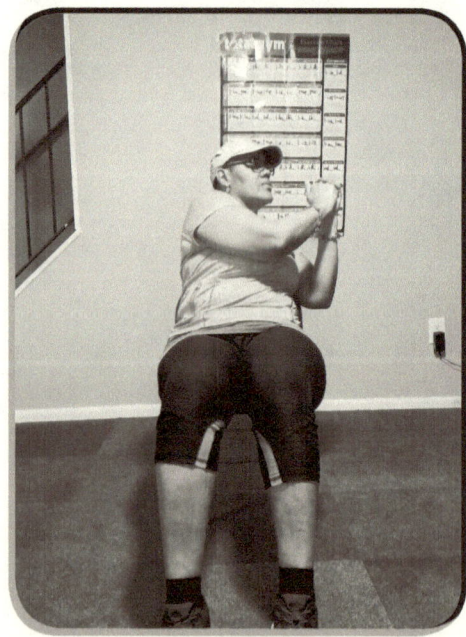

Russian Twist

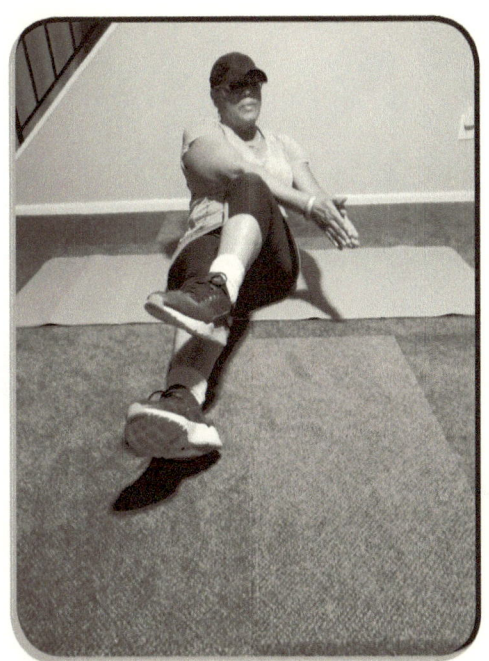

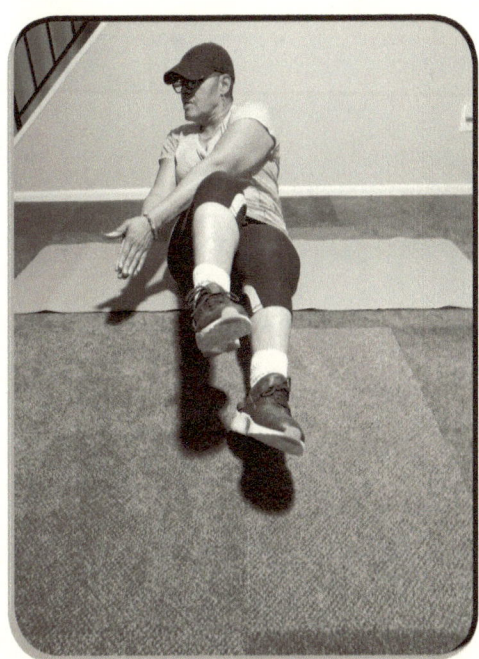

Cycling Russian Twist

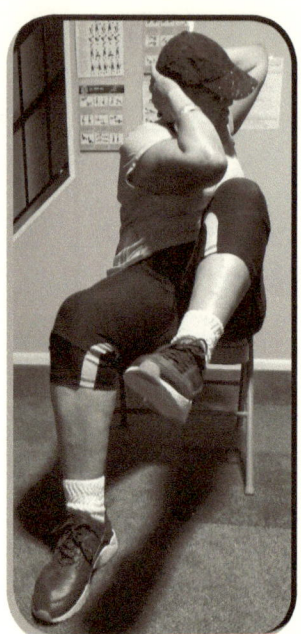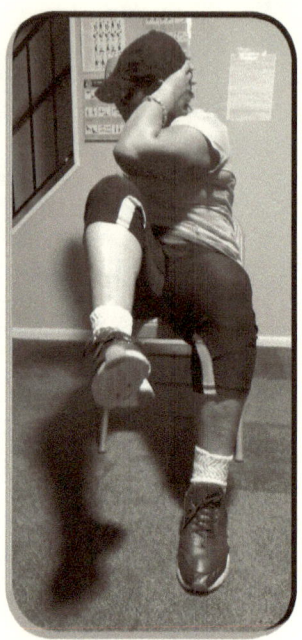

Knee to elbow lifts

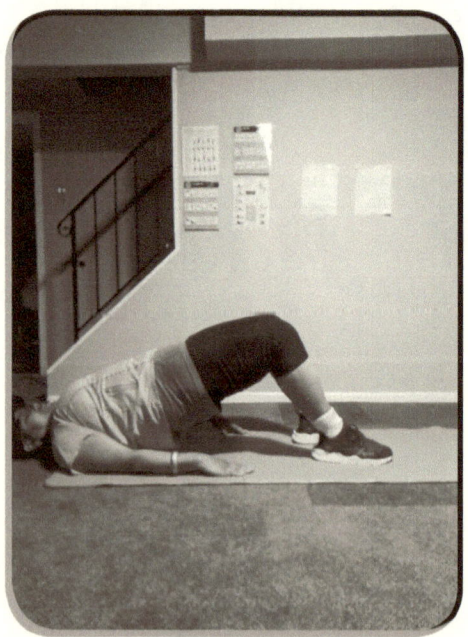

Hip bridge

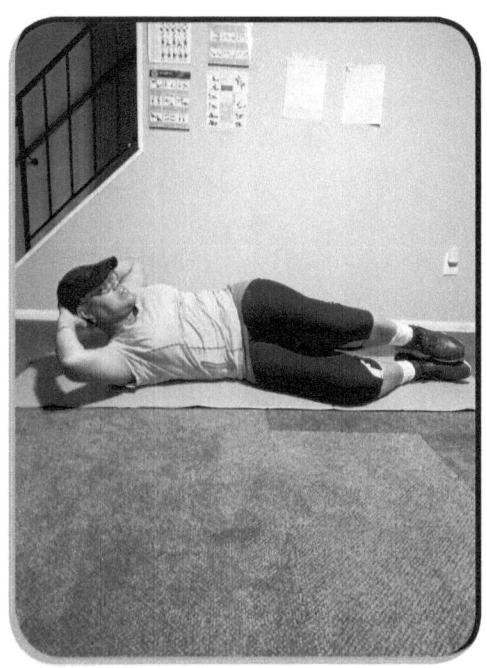

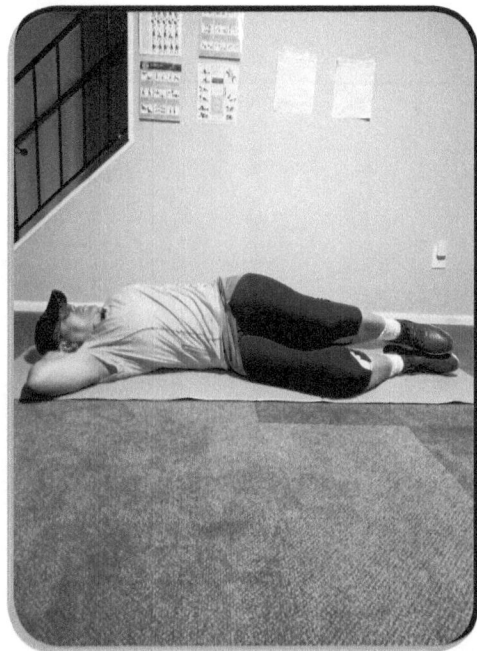

Side crunch

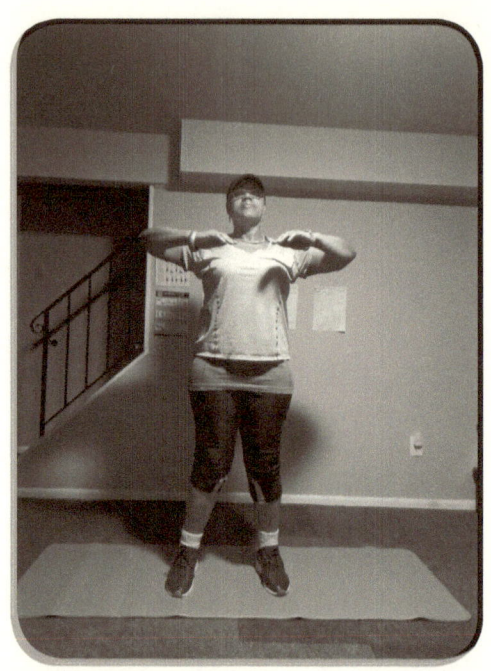

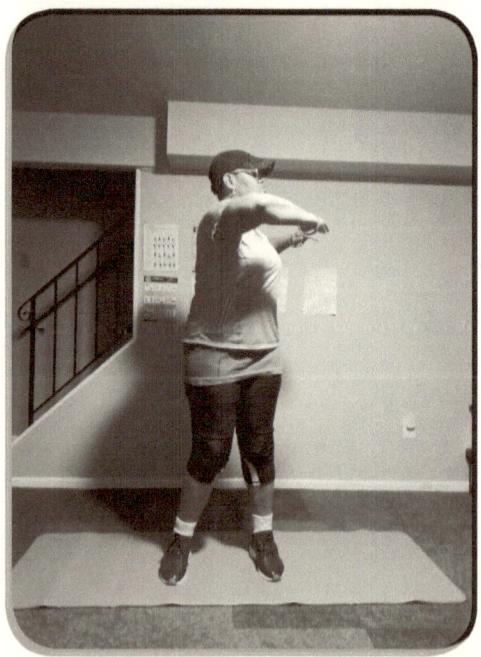

Side Twist

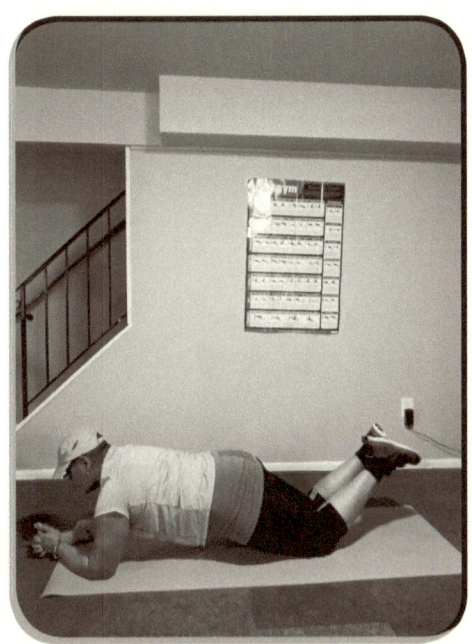

Plank one

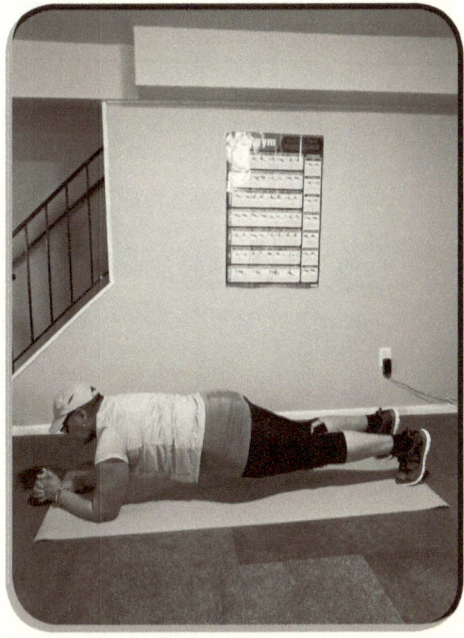

Plank two

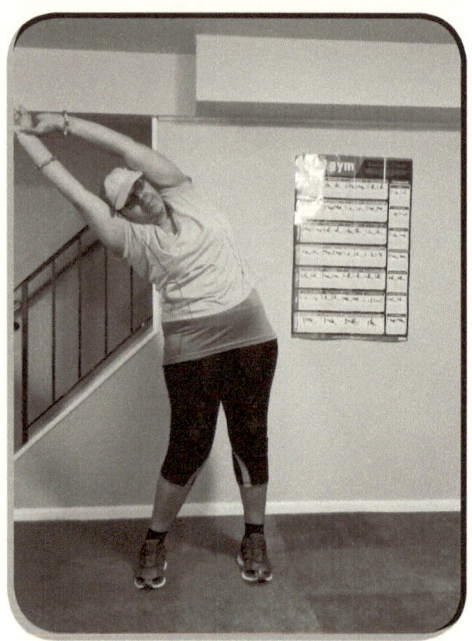

Arm side stretch

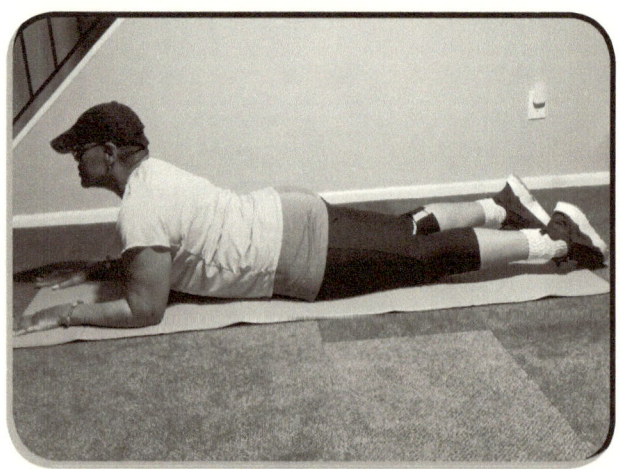

Beginning back bend #

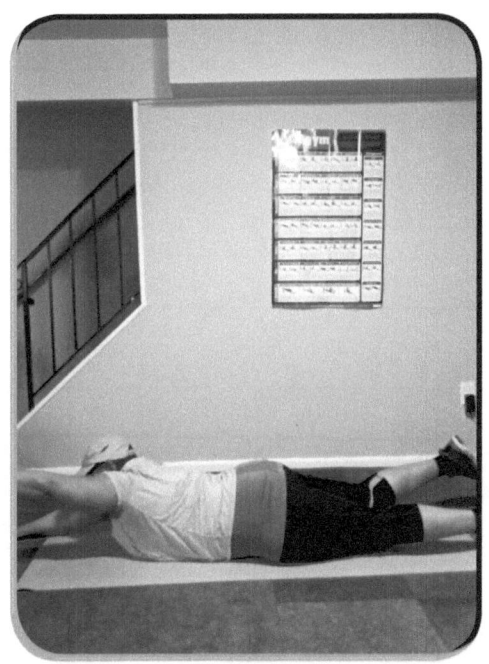

Superman hold

Notes

Notes

Notes

Notes

Notes

Notes

_____

_____

_____

_____

_____

_____

_____

_____

_____

_____

_____

_____

_____

_____

_____

Notes

Notes

Notes

_____

_____

_____

_____

_____

_____

_____

_____

_____

_____

_____

_____

_____

_____

Notes

_____

_____

_____

_____

_____

_____

_____

_____

_____

_____

_____

_____

_____

_____

_____

Notes

Notes

Notes

Notes

_____

_____

_____

_____

_____

_____

_____

_____

_____

_____

_____

_____

_____

_____

Notes

Notes

Notes

Notes

_____

_____

_____

_____

_____

_____

_____

_____

_____

_____

_____

_____

_____

_____

Notes

Notes

Notes

Notes

_____

_____

_____

_____

_____

_____

_____

_____

_____

_____

_____

_____

_____

_____

Notes

Notes

Notes

Notes

Notes

Notes

_____

_____

_____

_____

_____

_____

_____

_____

_____

_____

_____

_____

_____

Notes

_____

_____

_____

_____

_____

_____

_____

_____

_____

_____

_____

_____

_____

_____

Notes

Notes

Notes

Notes

Notes

Notes

Notes

Notes

Notes

Notes

Notes

Notes

Notes

Notes

Notes

Notes

Notes

_____

_____

_____

_____

_____

_____

_____

_____

_____

_____

_____

_____

_____

_____

Notes

Notes

Notes

Notes

Notes

Notes

Notes

Notes

Notes

Notes

Notes

Notes

Notes

Notes

Notes

_____

_____

_____

_____

_____

_____

_____

_____

_____

_____

_____

_____

_____

_____

Notes

www.ingramcontent.com/pod-product-compliance
Lightning Source LLC
Chambersburg PA
CBHW050408290526
45786CB00003B/1182